I0116810

Published in Great Britain by
L.R. Price Publications Ltd, 2022
27 Old Gloucester Street,
London, WC1N 3AX

www.lrpricepublications.com

ISBN: 9781915330376

Mindset and Health

Amira Elshalaby

I dedicate this book to all the people around the world who are seeking better health and life.

CONTENTS

INTRODUCTION

In this book, I will show how critical and lethal the state of mind is.

It is the key factor that determines illness or wellness; it can lead to either developing major diseases, aggravating pathogens and even death, or maintaining health and enhancing recovery.

The impact of a negative mental status on developing many physical health problems other than mental health problems not considered in this book is explained by how the psychological factor is greatly involved from contributing to developing many of the prevalent major chronic diseases such as cardiovascular diseases, stroke, and cancer. Also, how a negative mindset can worsen diseases, lead to catastrophic implications or even death.

Studies have revealed that people with a positive mindset never fall prey to despair or helplessness whether from illness or life situations and events which is the major cause of suicide, called death of despair.

Also, the impact of a positive mindset can prevent many diseases or reverse many of them. It also improves health as people who have a positive mindset always engage in healthy behaviours, habits and lifestyles that are critical for recovery and essential for enhancing health.

In addition, a positive mindset helps people avoid stress or even buffer its negative burden as they handle it proactively and positively.

Throughout this book, I am going to show how our thinking patterns interact with life events and circumstances. So, we deal with events as a result of our thinking patterns; we view, feel, decide, and act or behave to all life events and circumstances.

Therefore, our thinking patterns shape our personality traits, define who we are, how we perceive life, what kind of life we are going to have and live, and thus, of course, our health status.

I am going to reveal the relationship between mindset and health from a scientific point of view and the latest research standpoint in a simple, practical and detailed explanation including examples that are applicable in our everyday life with my own tiny hint or advice that might illuminate your vision to a healthy path.

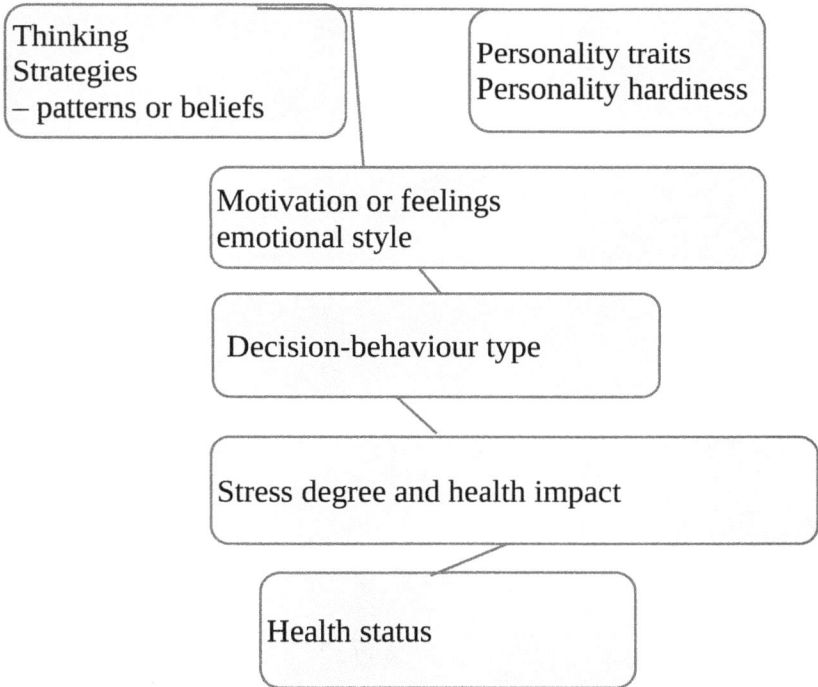

Thinking Strategies
– patterns or beliefs

Personality traits
Personality hardiness

Motivation or feelings emotional style

Decision-behaviour type

Stress degree and health impact

Health status

Let us begin our journey by discovering how we assess situations inside our minds and recognise the right approach to handle life events positively. And allow our minds to help us avoid stress and lead us towards health, as a negative mindset can be detrimental to our health and life.

PART 1: THINKING PATTERNS AND STRESS DEFINITION

FOCUS
- What is stress?
- Stress definition.
- Components of stress.
- What is meant by real stress?

What is stress?

The condition of stress has two components:

1. Physically involving direct material or bodily changes.
2. Psychologically involving how individuals perceive circumstances in their lives.

These components can be examined in three ways:

i. The first approach focuses on the environment. Stress is seen as a stimulus.

For example, when we have a demanding job or experience severe pain from a major disease, accident or death in the family.

Physically or psychologically challenging events or circumstances are called **stressors**.

ii. The second approach treats stress as a response focusing on people's reactions to stressors.

We see an example of this approach when people use the word stress to refer to their state of tension.
Our responses can be:

- o Psychological, for example, your thought pattern and emotions when you feel nervous, or angry.
- o Physiological, for example, when your heart pounds, your mouth goes dry and you perspire.

The psychological and physiological stressors are called **strains**.

iii. The third approach describes stress as a process that includes stressors and strains but adds an important dimension (the relationship between the person and the environment). This process involves continuous interactions and adjustments called **transactions** with the person and the environment each affecting and being affected by the other.
According to this view, stress is not just a stimulus or a response but rather a process in which the person is an active agent who can influence the impact of a stressor through behavioural, cognitive and emotional strategies that all stem from their well-held thinking strategies (beliefs) and the shape of their mind status (mindset).

For example, one person who is stuck in traffic and late for an important appointment keeps looking at their watch, honking their horn and getting angrier by the minute. Another person in the same circumstances stays calm, turns on the radio and listens to their favourite programs or songs.

Stress definition

Stress can be defined as the circumstance in which transactions lead a person to perceive a discrepancy between the physical or psychological demands of a situation and the resources of his or her biological, psychological or social systems.

Components of stress

Resources

Stress taxes the person's biopsychosocial resources with difficult events or circumstances. These resources are limited, thus one's resources are exposed to depletion as a result of trying to cope with their problems (they may need physical or psychiatric help). Sometimes, the impact is focused mainly on our biological system.

For example, when we tax our physical strength to lift something heavy.

More typically, however, the **strain** has an impact on all three systems and then becomes exhausted.

Demands

The phrase "demands of situation" refers to the amount of resources stress appears to require.

For example, one wants to lose weight so demands are as follows:

- o Stop eating junk foods and sweet drinks.
- o Exercise regularly.
- o Avoid alcohol and cigarettes.

Discrepancy

When there is a poor fit or a mismatch between the demands of the situation and the resources of the person, a discrepancy exists. This generally has taken the form of the demands taxing or exceeding the resources.

For example, when someone wants to lose weight but feels they do not have the willpower to restrict their diet or exercise regularly.

But the opposite discrepancy also occurs, that is, our resources may be underutilised and this can be stressful too. A worker or employer who is bored by a lack of challenge in a job may find this situation stressful.

Transaction

In our transaction with the environment, we assess demands, resources and discrepancies between them.
These transactions are affected by many factors including our prior experience and aspects of the current situations.

An important point to keep in mind is that a demand, resource or discrepancy may be either real or just believed to exist.

For example, suppose you had taken a major exam and wanted to do well but worried greatly that you would not. If you had procrastinated and did not prepare well for the test, the discrepancy you see between the demands and your resources might be real. But, if you had previously done well on similar exams, prepared well enough for this one, and scored well on a pre-test in a study guide yet still thought you would not do well, the discrepancy you see would not reflect the true state of affairs.

Stress often results from inaccurate perceptions of discrepancies between environmental demands and actual resources. Stress is in the eye of the beholder, which emphasises the importance of accurate perception and precise assessment of situations or events so as to not fall prey to stress that could not exist.

Therefore, I referred to it as "avoid stress" in the introduction of the book. This means we can also avoid a lot of stress that is untrue.

For example, you may have symptoms of nausea, vomiting, and mild fever, as you are saturated with news of Covid-19 symptoms. So, if you did not stay calm and rational, you would jump to the conclusion that you have Covid-19, you would experience great stress, be so panicked, and try to self-medicate, which may worsen your symptoms or even more dangerously, hurt your health condition thus of course leading to more panic.

Such a vicious cycle and its negative consequences or hazards could be halted if you stayed quiet, rational and sought medical supervision and never jump into foolish assumptions about your symptoms. In this way, you would save your health and yourself from mental torture.

PART 2: THINKING PATTERNS AND ASSESSMENT OF EVENTS

FOCUS

- How our perception and interpretation of events are the key determinants as to whether the event is stressful or not to us.
- What are primary and secondary appraisals?
- Cognition and stress two-way communication.
- Coping with stress.
- What other factors lead to stressful appraisals?

How our perception and interpretation of events are the key determinants as to whether the event is stressful or not to us

This clarifies that mind status is the key factor to determine health. Let us see how.

Transactions in stress generally involve an assessment process that researchers Richard Lazarus et al called **cognitive appraisal**, which is a mental process by which people assess two factors:

1. Whether a demand threatens their physical or psychological wellbeing.
2. The resources available for meeting the demand.

These are called primary and secondary appraisals.

What are primary and secondary appraisals?

Primary appraisal

For example, when we experience symptoms of pain or nausea, we first try to assess the meaning of the situation for our wellbeing. This assessment process is called primary appraisal.

This appraisal seeks answers to questions such as "What does this mean to me?" and "Will I be okay or in trouble?" Your primary appraisal regarding pain or nausea could yield one of three judgments:

1. **It is irrelevant:** you might decide this if you had similar symptoms of pain and nausea before that lasted only a short while and were not followed by illness.

2. **It is good:** this is called benign positive, which might be your appraisal if you really wanted to skip work or have a college exam postponed.

3. **It is stressful:** you might decide this if you feared the symptoms were of a serious illness such as a cancerous tumour that might be a life-threatening type.

Circumstances we appraise as stressful receive further appraisal for three implications:

1. **Harm loss:** this refers to the amount of damage that has already occurred when someone is incapacitated and in pain following a serious injury.

Sometimes, people who experience a relatively minor stressor think of it as a disaster thereby exaggerating its personal impact and increasing their feelings of stress.

2. **Threat:** this involves the expectation of future harm.

For example, when one is exposed to a critical illness, they begin to worry about medical costs, difficult rehabilitation, expected pain or restriction and loss of income and the consequences.
Stress appraisals seem to depend heavily on harm loss and threat.

3. **Challenge:** this is the opportunity to achieve growth, mastery, or profit by using more than routine resources to meet a demand.

For example, when one is faced with a period of illness that may demand staying at home for a long time, they could make it a way to increase their knowledge, and skills, and improve their health with diet or exercise and spiritual practices. So, as they end their recovery period, they are able to have higher payments for their job or may be able to get another job as they have raised their skills.
They also get to live happier and stronger as they have enhanced their mental, physical and spiritual health thus also, affecting their social life positively and guaranteeing happiness. Instead of other people who make their life seem like hell by facing the fact of being sick.

Secondary appraisal

This refers to our assessment of the resources we have available for coping, although these assessments occur continuously in our transactions. We are especially aware of secondary appraisals when we judge a situation as potentially stressful and try to determine whether our resources are sufficient to meet the harm, threat, or challenge we face.

The condition of stress that we experience often depends on the outcome of the appraisal we make. When we judge that our resources are sufficient to meet the demands, we may experience little or no stress, but when we appraise demands as greater than our resources, we may feel a great deal of stress.

These processes determine everyday stress responses, but also influence much more severe reactions such as the development of a serious disorder (if such negative thinking patterns become permanent and habitual).

Cognition and stress two-way communication

Stress can impair cognitive functioning by distracting our attention.

For example, when one has a sad event or illness of someone close to them, they might try to distract themselves by focusing their attention on other things. As a result, when they are confronted at work or school with even a simple question, they would not be able to give an accurate answer, which means that such a stressful event has impaired their cognition.

Also, studies revealed that noise can be a stressor that can be chronic for people who live in a noisy environment like next to a railroad. Many try to deal with it by changing the focus of their attention from the noise to relevant aspects of a cognitive task and as a result, they tune out the noise.

Evidence suggests that children who try to tune out chronic noise may develop generalised cognitive deficits because they have difficulty knowing which sound to attend to and which to tune out. Not only can stress affect cognition, but the reverse is true too.

For example, worrying about future threats and ruminating about past difficulties can maintain elevated physiological stress responses even in the absence of actual stressful situations.

The two-way connection between cognition and stress is particularly important in the group of cognitive processes called **executive functioning**. This refers to a set of cognitive abilities involved in the regulation and direction of our ongoing behaviour such as maintaining and shifting attention as needed, inhibiting unhelpful or inappropriate responses or impulses, and selecting among alternative responses under consideration.

These are the cognitive processes that enable us to direct or guide our behaviour intentionally. Better executive cognitive functioning can obviously help one manage the demands of stressful situations but stressful experiences can also temporarily deplete or fatigue these cognitive resources.

Depleted executive cognitive resources can lead to more difficulty dealing with stressful situations, creating a possible vicious cycle of stress and impaired cognition.

The same aspects of cognitive functioning are supported by structures and circuits in the pre-frontal cortex of the brain that also support parasympathetic "brakes" on physiological stress responses.

So, difficulties thinking clearly during stress might be accompanied by poor physiological control or regulation of the stress response.

Cognition and emotions related to stress

Emotions tend to accompany stress and people often use their emotional states to evaluate their stress which depends on a cognitive appraisal to stress.

For example, one might experience fear if they assess a situation as being a threat, (for example, seeing a snake in a room) and might experience anxiety if they assess that the situation is not familiar to them (for example, a patient awaiting surgery). Also, one might experience a feeling of sadness or even anger according to one's cognitive appraisals.

We are all humans experiencing stress and trying to deal with it. So, let us see the importance of coping with stress.

Coping with stress

What is really meant by coping with stress? Is there positive and negative coping?

It is the process by which people try to manage the perceived discrepancy between the demands of the situation and the resources they appraise in a stressful situation. Manage in definition indicates that coping efforts can be quite varied and do not necessarily lead to a solution to the problem.

Although coping efforts can be aimed at correcting or mastering the problem, they may also help the perception of a discrepancy, to tolerate or accept the harm or threat, or escape or avoid the situation.

We cope with stress through our cognitive and behavioural transactions with the environment.

For example, if a man's doctor asked him to quit smoking or lose weight as such factors endanger his heart health, this presents a threat to him as he may become disabled or die. And it is stressful especially if he could not change his behaviour. How can he cope with this?

The answer is, he can cope with this in either a negative or a positive way according to his mindset (thinking pattern or style).

So, he can cope with this positively, by seeking information about ways to improve his ability to change. Positive coping is always referred to as **problem-focused coping** and is aimed at reducing the demands of a stressful situation or expanding the resources to deal with it.

Of course, by coping positively the person allows his mind to decide rationally and thus act or behave wisely which in turn improves his heart health, saves his life and consequently has a better social life. On the other hand, he may cope negatively, by refusing to change his habits and simply finding another doctor that is not so directive or by simply referring habitual change to God's hands. The one who acts negatively threatens their health and life thus impairing their social life.

Negative coping sometimes referred to as **emotion-focused coping**, is aimed at controlling the emotional response to a stressful situation. People tend to use emotion-focused approaches when they believe they can do little to change a stressful situation, such as the death of a close person. People can regulate their emotional responses through **behavioural-cognitive** approaches.

Examples of behavioural approaches can be healthy or unhealthy, such as:

1. Using alcohol or drugs.
2. Seeking emotional social support from friends or relatives.
3. Engaging in activities like sports or watching TV that distracts attention from the problem.

Examples of cognitive approaches involve how people think about a stressful situation, such as redefining the situation and trying to put a good face on it. People who want to redefine a stressful situation can generally find a way to do it since there is almost always some aspect of one's life that can be viewed positively.
Other emotion-focused cognitive processes include **defence mechanisms** that involve distorting memory or

reality in some way. One defence mechanism is called **denial**.

In serious medical situations, people who are diagnosed with terminal diseases often use this strategy and refuse to believe they are ill. This is one way by which people cope by using avoidance strategies. Such strategies can be helpful in the short run like during an early stage of a prolonged stress experience, thereafter, coping is better served by giving the situation attention.

People tend to use emotion-focused approaches when they believe they can do little to change a stressful situation, for example, when a loved one dies. In this situation, people often seek emotional support and distract themselves with being involved in funeral issues and house chores or work demands.

Note: coping methods that focus on emotions are critical because sometimes they interfere with getting medical treatment or involve unhealthy behaviours like using cigarettes, alcohol or drugs to reduce tension.

This reveals again the importance of rational thinking or mindset as it not only helps prevent stress but, also helps cope with it in order to assess it in a firm, quick and healthy approach thus, enhancing one's health and life as well as the health and welfare of those who surround them.

<u>What other factors lead to stressful appraisals?</u>

Appraising events as stressful depends on two types of factors, those related to the person and those related to the situation.

Personal factors

These include intellectual, motivational and personality characteristics.

One example is self-esteem. People who have high self-esteem are likely to believe that they have sources to meet demands that require the strengths they possess. If they perceive an event as stressful. They may interpret it as a challenge rather than a threat.

Another example relates to motivation. The more important a threatened goal, the more stress the person is likely to perceive.

One other example involves the person's belief system, as psychologist Albert Ellis has noted, many people have irrational beliefs that increase their stress, for instance, because one strongly desires to have a safe, comfortable and satisfying life:

"The conditions under which I live absolutely must be easy, peaceful and gratifying and this one I am facing is awful and I cannot bear it and I cannot be happy at all when they are unsafe and frustrating."

A person who holds such a belief is likely to appraise almost any sort of inconvenience as harmful or threatening. The tendency to appraise even minor issues as major problems is often called perfectionism and this thinking style not only causes emotional distress but can also pose a serious threat to long-term health.

Situational factors

If the event involves very strong demands and is imminent, the situation tends to be seen as stressful, which makes the situation really stressful.

For example, patients who expect to undergo a physically uncomfortable or painful medical procedure tomorrow, are likely to view their situation as being more stressful than say, expecting to have a blood pressure test next week.

Let us recognise the characteristics of stressful situations.

Life transitions

Passing from one life condition to another, for example, retiring from a career.

Difficult timing

Events that happen earlier or later in life than usual or expected, for example, having a baby in old age, you are not even expecting it and the baby's health condition is not well.

Ambiguity

A lack of clarity in a situation, for example, unclear information about job performance.

Low desirability

Some circumstances are undesirable to most people in virtually all respects, for example, losing your wallet somewhere outside.

Low controllability

Circumstances that seem to be outside the person's behavioural or cognitive influence, for example, a close person to you has a deep problem and there is nothing you can do to help them, or maybe you do not have the appropriate strategies to help them.

Research revealed that the amount of stress a person experiences increases with stress or frequency, intensity and duration. Evidence supports this assumption that the stronger the stressors, the greater the physiological strain.

Let us see the stress effects on the body.

PART 3: STRESS EFFECTS ON THE BODY

FOCUS
- Body response to stress and biological response to stress.
- What is meant by physiological arousal?
- Factors that determine body response to stress.

Body response to stress and biological aspects of stress

The physiological portion of the response to a stressor or strain is called **reactivity**, which researchers measure by comparison against a baseline or resting level of arousal.

1. Genetic factors influence people's degree of reactivity to stressors.

2. People who are under chronic stress often show heightened reactivity when a stressor occurs and their arousal may take more time to return to baseline levels.

A famous researcher (Walter Cannon, 1929) provided a basic description of how the body reacts to emergencies. This reaction has been called **fight or flight response** because it prepares the organism to attack the threat or flee. In the fight or flight response, the perception of danger causes the sympathetic nervous system to stimulate many organs like the heart directly and stimulate the adrenal glands of the endocrine system which secrete epinephrine arousing the body further still.

Cannon proposed that this arousal could have positive or negative effects. The fight or flight response is adaptive because it mobilises the organism to respond quickly to danger, but this high arousal can be harmful to health if prolonged.

What is meant by physiological arousal?

The effects of the body having to adapt repeatedly to stressors such as fluctuation in levels of hormones like cortisol and epinephrine, blood pressure and immune function that accumulate over time are called **allostatic load**, which creates wear and tear on the body and impairs its ability to adapt to future stressors.

Studies of chronic stress have confirmed that high levels of allostatic load are related to poor health in children and the elderly. Its concept highlights the importance of considering the overall accumulation of physiological strains over time.

The cumulative amount of strain typically has a greater influence on health than the degree of activation in response to any stressors.

Factors that determine body response to stress

The following four factors are important in the overall amount of bodily activation or physiological stress:

1. **Amount of exposure:** this is obviously key – when we encounter more frequent, intense or prolonged stressors, we are likely to respond in a greater amount of physiological activation.

2. **Magnitude of reactivity:** in response to any particular stressor, such as taking a major academic exam, some individuals will show a large increase in blood pressure or stress hormones while others will show much smaller changes.

3. **Rate of recovery:** once the encounter with a stressor is over, physiological responses return to normal quickly for some people, but stay elevated for a longer time for others who continue to think about the stressor after it is over, revisiting it mentally, or worrying about it.

Recurrence in the future can delay physiological recovery and add to the accumulated toll through prolonged physiological activation.

4. **Resource restoration:** The resources used in physiological strain are replenished by various activities and sleep may be the most important of them. Sleep deprivation can be a source of stress and contributes to allostatic load directly.

In addition, poor sleep quality or reduced amounts of sleep predict the development of serious health problems, such as heart disease. During sleep, some aspects of physiological activity typically drop below daytime levels similar to what happens with blood pressure. The larger the drop, the more beneficial for health, but this can be disrupted by daily stressors.

The restoration of stress resources has a major impact on allostatic load and related health consequences.

Note: Sleeping is crucial to reverse stress's negative health impacts. Also, sleeping is just as important as nutrition and exercise to your health and bodily functions and body composition as well as your performance.

Good sleep helps our bodies and minds recover, and keeps us lean, happy, mentally focused and healthy. However, chronically bad sleep increases our body fat ratio, disturbs our hormones, speeds up the ageing process, makes our mental effort or power fade and depletes our energy and joy resources.

New research found that when healthy men in their 20s got only five hours of sleep per night, the way their bodies metabolised fat shifted. Rather than evaporating triglyceride-rich lipoproteins that have been linked to the formation of clogging and dangerous fatty plaques in the arteries, their bodies began storing them.

Research showed that:

1. Sleep deprivation over a period of time has been linked to several serious health conditions including hypertension, obesity, diabetes, and a suppressed immune system.

2. Not getting enough sleep has a significant impact on our day-to-day and long-term health.

3. It has been well documented that getting adequate sleep helps strengthen our immune system and is

associated with a decreased risk of cardiovascular and metabolic diseases, including obesity and type 2 diabetes.

4. One such way sleep deprivation hurts us, is that it makes us feel less full even after eating a high-fat dinner.

A study recently published in the Journal of Lipid Research addressed how getting five hours of sleep a night, four days a week followed by one 10-hour night of "recovery sleep" affected 15 healthy men in their 20s. Specifically, how it affected their postprandial lipemia or the rise of triglyceride-rich lipoproteins.

What the researchers found was not good: "The lipids weren't evaporating – they were being stored." Experts assure us that lack of sleep makes our jobs more stressful.

The results were nearly identical for men and women, but some races and professions were getting hit harder than others in the US study.

Also, research revealed that not getting enough sleep can affect the way we think and react, which includes decreased alertness and memory impairment, and that poor sleep also affects our mood. Over a long period of time, more hours of lost rest increase a person's risk of accidents and overall poor quality of life.

Lack of good sleep can translate to not only obesity and diabetes, but also high blood pressure, a suppressed immune system, low sex drive, and an overall chance of death apart from any other medical condition. Mentally that can lead to anxiety, depression, paranoia, and even hallucinations. Even in children, studies revealed that a lack of sleep can lead to hyperactivity, which could be confused with attention deficit hyperactivity disorder (ADHD).

In addition, research showed that adequate sleep is even more important than adequate eating or exercising to maintain our overall health. Fortunately, research assured that returning to adequate sleep can quickly reduce the risks.

Thus, it is important to always adhere to healthy methods and practices throughout the day to keep you calm, and rational, and be able to help you have a good sleep in the quantity of seven to nine hours a day, and more importantly in the quality.

Examples of these healthy practices during the daytime:

1. Walking for 30-60 minutes daily.

2. Avoiding alcohol.

3. Restricting to a healthy diet rich in these food types: complex carbohydrates (such as wholegrains, sweet potatoes, brown rice and pasta), lean meat, fresh vegetables, legumes, and yoghurt. Avoid food high in sugar and fat, processed meat and processed foods. It is better to eat nuts and fruits to boost your mood.

It is also OK to eat a small portion of high nutritional value sweets, for instance, cakes, biscuits or ice cream if this would help you to restrict your healthy routine, if not, you had better adhere to fruits only or some nuts.

4. Limit caffeine consumption, especially before bedtime.

5. Meditation and yoga.

6. Always seek social support.

7. Engage in useful or joyful activities.

8. Make a daily sleep routine for sleeping and waking up.

Studies say, "It's harder for the brain to turn off" and "Let the mind have time to wind down." Therefore, it is recommended to avoid those glowing screens an hour – two, ideally – before bedtime. But, using technology by setting a sleep alarm telling you it is time to climb into a comfortable bed in a dark, quiet room is one way to use technology to help you sleep.

9. Always have a rational talk with yourself at the end of the day to assess your problems realistically, and make wise decisions in a reasonable and systematic plan. Before you go to sleep you can read a book or listen to relaxing music.

As we have just seen, four factors determine our physiological responses to stress burden. Research assures that the increased physiological responses to stressors (the greater reactivity, the more delayed the recovery, and the reduced resources restoration) worsen or even endanger health status.

Some studies revealed that chronic worrying or ruminating events whether they are major or simple could be associated with Alzheimer's or dementia. Some study authors found that older adults who regularly engaged in what is called repetitive thinking were more likely to experience cognitive decline including memory problems than those who did not. They also had higher levels of the proteins beta-amyloid and tau in their brains.

The accumulation of these proteins which create damaging clumps known as plaques and tangles in the brain is a hallmark of Alzheimer's that begins in the earliest stages of the disease even before an individual experiences visible symptoms of dementia.

PART 4: PERSONAL BELIEFS, PERSONALITY TRAITS AND STRESS

FOCUS

- Why does stress lead to illness in some individuals, but not in others? What is the diathesis-stress model?
- What factors are involved in developing stress that leads to illness?
- Personality traits lead to behaviours thus defining stress, therefore, health status.
- Beliefs about oneself and feelings of personal control reduce the stress people experience.
- How people develop personal control.
- Feelings of lack of personal control and health consequences.

Why does stress lead to illness in some individuals, but not in others? What is the diathesis-stress model?

There is one answer: other factors influence the effects of stress. This idea forms the basis of the **diathesis-stress model** which explains that people's vulnerability to a physical or psychological disorder depends on the interplay of their predisposition to the disorder **diathesis** and the amount of stress they experience.

The predisposition can result from an organic structure and functioning often genetically determined, or from prior environmental conditions, such as living in a community that promotes tobacco use.

For example, chronically high levels of stress are especially likely to lead to chronic heart disease if the person's body produces high levels of cholesterol. Or students are likely to catch a cold during major exams if their immune system functioning is impaired. This concept may explain why not all individuals in the following experiment caught a cold.

Researchers conducted an interesting experiment. They gave people nasal drops that contained either a common cold virus or a placebo solution and then quarantined them to check for infection and cold symptoms.

Before the nasal drops were administered, the subjects filled out a questionnaire to assess their recent stress. Of these people, 47% of those with high stress and 27% of those with low stress developed colds. Other studies have produced three related findings:

- **First**, people under chronic severe stress are more vulnerable to catching a cold when exposed to the virus than people under less stress.

- **Second**, people who experience a lot of positive emotions, such as feeling energetic or happy are less likely to catch a cold when exposed to the virus than people who have fewer of these emotions.

- **Third**, people who have sleep problems prior to their exposure to the virus are more likely to develop colds.

What factors are involved in developing stress that leads to illness?

The casual consequence can involve two routes:

1. A direct route resulting from changes stress produces in the body's physiology.

2. An indirect route affecting health through the person's behaviour.

Personality traits lead to behaviours thus defining stress, therefore, health status

Behaviour that is the result of mindset or beliefs which in turn determine stress, affect in either negative or positive way thus, health status.

We can see the behavioural links between stress and illness in many stressful situations. People who experience high levels of stress tend to behave in ways that increase their chances of becoming ill or injured. For instance, compared with people with low stress, people with high stress are more likely to eat high-fat diets with fewer fruits and vegetables, engage in less exercise, smoke cigarettes and consume more alcohol.

These behaviours are associated with the development of various illnesses. In addition, stress impairs sleep. And the resulting inattention and carelessness probably play a role in the relatively high accident rates of people under stress.

Studies revealed that children and adults who experience high levels of stress are more likely to suffer accidental injuries at home, in sports activities, on the job and while driving cars than individuals under less stress. Further, disrupted sleep can itself be stressful and as known, poor sleep prominently interferes with the way that the body is restored physiologically.

Now we will see the role of mindset or beliefs which is the root of behaviour in influencing stress in either a positive or negative way. Personality traits stem from the mindset and affect one's feelings, decision-making, and actions or behaviour, which in turn can increase or decrease stress.

One important factor that modifies the stress people experience is the degree of control people feel they have in their lives. Thus, people strive for a sense of **personal control**; the feeling that they can make decisions and take effective actions to produce desirable outcomes and avoid undesirable ones.

Studies have found that people who have a strong sense of personal control report experiencing less strain from stressors.

<u>Beliefs about oneself and feelings of personal control reduce the stress people experience</u>

People can use several types of control to influence events in their lives and reduce their stress. I am going to focus on two aspects:

1. Behavioural control involves the ability to take concrete action to reduce the impact of stressors. This action might reduce the intensity of the event or shorten its duration.

For example, a pregnant woman who has taken natural childbirth classes can use special breathing techniques during delivery that reduce the pain of labour.

For example, a person is going to perform a public speech so they took in advance many courses for such a performance, and then they trained in situations that mimic the public speech. Thus, they are able to control their anxiety before and during the speech also, increasing or even assuring their chance of success.

2. Cognitive control is the ability to use thought processes or strategies to modify the impact of a stressor, such as by thinking about the event differently or focusing on a pleasant or neutral thought. Cognitive reappraisal of stressful stimuli or events is less threatening and can reduce negative emotions and physiological stress responses.

For example, when you are dieting you may feel stressed, angry or even frustrated as you feel hungry or are doing more exercises or even limiting or avoiding your previous delicious, unhealthy eating habits. Therefore, if you rethink your condition and see that you are preventing disease, optimising your wellness, and losing weight thus regaining your fit shape and imagining the healthier, more beautiful version of you, in this way you make stress fade and be more encouraged to keep on track.

For example, while pregnant, the mother might think about the positive meanings the baby will give to her life, or she could focus her mind on an image such as a joyful day she had at a picnic.

Cognitive control appears to be especially effective in reducing stress.

People differ in the degree to which they believe as to whether they have control over their own lives. People who believe they have control over their successes and failures are described as possessing an **internal locus of control**. That is the control for the events that lie within themselves; they are responsible.

Other people who believe that their lives are controlled by forces outside of themselves, for example, by luck, have an **external locus of control**.

For the importance of personal control degree, there is a questionnaire called the I-E Scale, which is used to measure the degree of the internality or externality of a person's beliefs about personal control. Another important aspect of personal control is our sense of **self-efficacy**: the belief that we can succeed at a specific activity we want to do.

People estimate their chances of success at any goal, such as in academic achievement, or in an activity such as quitting smoking. Based on their prior observations of themselves and others, they decide whether to attempt the activity according to two expectations:

1. **Outcome expectancy:** the behaviour, if properly carried out, would lead to a favourable outcome.

2. **Self-efficacy expectancy:** they can perform the behaviour properly.

For example, you may know that by taking and doing well in a set of college honours courses you can graduate with a special diploma or certificate. But, if you think the likelihood of achieving that feat is improbable, you are not likely to try.

So, for people engaged in a stressful activity, and experiencing an increased heart rate and blood pressure, generally, this is due to their level of mental effort in dealing with the demands of the situation.
"The greater their effort, the greater cardiovascular reactivity."

Thus, people with strong efficacy for the activity may be less threatened and exert less mental effort because they know they can manage the demands of the situation more easily. Hence, they generally show less psychological and physiological strain than those with weaker self-efficacy.

Now, it has been made clear what is meant by personal control's impact on stress degree thus, health status.

How people develop personal control

We make these assessments by:

a. Using the information we gain from our experiences, successes and failures throughout life.

b. Our **sense of control** also developed through social learning in which we learn by observing the behaviour of others.

For example, during childhood, people in the family and at school are important to others, serving as models of behaviour, agents of reinforcement and standards for comparison. At the other end of the life span, people tend to be relatively external in the locus of control that is, the beliefs that chance and powerful people affect their lives are greater in the elderly than in younger adults.

So, among older adults, when faced with a serious illness or problem, they are more inclined to prefer having professionals make health-related decisions for them.

<u>Feelings of lack of personal control and health consequences</u>

What happens to people who experience high levels of stress over a long period and feel that nothing they do matters? They feel helpless, trapped and unable to avoid negative outcomes.

This condition is called **learned helplessness**, which describes a principal characteristic of depression. Research has shown that people can learn to be helpless by being in uncontrollable situations that lead to repeated failure. Researchers Seligman et al have extended the theory of learned helplessness to explain two important observations:

- **First**, being exposed to uncontrollable, negative events does not always lead to learned helplessness.

- **Second**, depressed people often report feeling a loss in self-esteem. The revised theory proposes that people who experience uncontrollable negative events apply a cognitive process called **attribution** in which they make judgments about three dimensions of the situation. As in the following:

1. **Internal-external**: people consider whether the situation results from their own personality's inability to control outcomes or from external causes that are beyond anyone's control.

2. **Stable-unstable**: People assess whether the situation results from a cause that is long-lasting (stable) or temporary (unstable). If they judge that is long-lasting, for example, when people develop a chronic and disabling disease, they are more likely to feel helpless and depressed than if they think their condition is temporary.

3. **Global-specific**: people consider whether the situation results from factors that have global and wide-ranging effects or specific and narrow effects.

Example for global judgment: someone may feel helpless and depressed, "I am totally not good and do not amount to anything."

Example for specific judgment: others who fail and make a specific judgment, such as "I am not good at controlling this part of my life", are less likely to feel helpless.

Further example: If you have experienced an unfair deal within one company in a certain city or region, people with **global** judgment will say, "This company is no good, I will never trust them or work with this company and any other one in this city or region." However, **specific** ones would consider the reasons and see if the company has any excuses, they would stop working with them or lose trust in it and never create an accurate conclusion about all the companies in the whole city or region unless he found real accurate data or evidence.

Thus, people who tend to attribute negative events in their lives to stable and global causes are at a high risk of feeling helpless and depressed. If their judgments are also internal, their depressive thinking is likely to include a loss of self-esteem as well.

People who believe bad events result from internal, stable global factors while good events result from external, unstable and specific factors have a pessimistic explanatory style.

For example, if someone faced failure in their business, people with a pessimistic explanatory style would say, "I am such a failure, I do not amount to anything, I am always out of luck, maybe this business is no good for anyone. I am always destined by miseries and catastrophes."

Attributing negative events to external, unstable, specific causes, in contrast, reflects an optimistic explanatory or attributional style.

For example, people with an optimistic explanatory or attributional style would say when faced with the same failure in business that firstly, they accept failures as a natural part of life as well as successes. They try to figure out the reasons, assess their work trying to consider improvements, better plans, and smarter efforts. If they found that things were out of their control, they would accept this proudly as a failure that was not their fault.

Evidence reveals that **lacking personal control** affects people negatively in real-life stressful conditions. Studies have examined this conclusion with college students and children.

For instance, of college students in dormitories, those who lived on crowded floors reported more stress and less ability to control unwanted social interaction and showed more evidence of helplessness such as "giving up in competitive games, than those on uncrowded floors."

In a study of fifth graders, students were given the impossible task of arranging blocks to match a pictured design. Children who attributed their failure to stable, uncontrollable factors, such as their own lack of ability, showed poorer performance on subsequent problems than those who attributed the failure to unstable, modified factors, such as lack of effort.

Thus, the children's attributions were linked to their feelings of helplessness.

Personal control positive impact on health

There are two ways in which personal control and health may be related. First, people who have a strong sense of personal control may be more likely or able to maintain their health and prevent illness than those who have a weak sense of control. Second, once people become seriously ill, those who have a strong sense of control may adjust to the illness and promote their own rehabilitation better than those who have a weak sense of control.

Both types of relationships have been studied. In order to study these relationships, researchers have used several approaches to measure people's control.

One of the best-developed health-related measures of personal control is the Multidimensional Health Locus of Control Scales. This instrument contains 18 items divided into three scales that assess:

1. **Internal health locus of control**. The belief is that the control over one's health lies within the person.

2. **Powerful other health locus of control**. The belief is that one's health is controlled by other people such as physicians.

3. **Chance locus of control**. The belief that luck or fate controls health.

The sense of personal control influences people's health significantly in either a positive or negative way.

Studies have shown that pessimistic and hopeless people who believe they have little control, have poorer health habits, more illnesses and are less likely to take active steps to treat their illnesses than people with a greater sense of control.

Studies also revealed that personal control can help people adjust to becoming seriously ill. Patients with illnesses such as kidney failure or a critical cancer type, who score high on internal locus of control, suffer less depression than those with strong beliefs in the role of chance.

The belief that either they, someone else or even something else (e.g., something they believe in or merely abstract positive belief) can influence the course of their illness allows patients to be hopeful about their future. Moreover, patients with a strong internal locus of control beliefs probably realise they have effective ways of controlling their stress.

Personal control also affects the efforts patients make toward rehabilitation, in particular, feelings of self-efficacy enhance their efforts.

For example, a study demonstrated this with older adult patients who had serious respiratory diseases such as chronic bronchitis and emphysema. The patients were examined at a clinic and given individualised prescriptions for exercise. They rated on a survey their self-efficacy, that is, their belief in their ability to perform specific physical activity, such as:

    a. Walking different distances.
    b. Lifting objects of various weights.
    c. Climbing stairs.

Correlation analysis revealed that the greater the patient's self-efficacy for doing physical activity, the more they adhered to the exercise prescription.

Health hint: Many studies revealed that the more active we are, the greater our self-esteem is, and the happier, more intelligent, and more communicative we are. Even if such activities are so simple like the following daily life activities:
- Going to the supermarket and doing household chores.
- Gardening.
- Walking with your pets.
- Pulling or dragging things like a heavy door.
- Stepping over obstacles.

Being physically active improves our cognitive ability (thinking, remembering, learning).

Research indicates a theory called **embodied cognition** in which the body's movements influence brain functioning like processing information, decision making, and vice versa.

Let me explain.

Since movement resides in our entire body and it is known that thinking is limited to the brain, there is evidence that movement and thoughts are the two sides of the same coin. It turns out that the cerebellum (a structure at the base of the brain) in the past was thought to be responsible for only balance, posture, muscle coordination and motor skills. Now, its role in thinking and emotions has been vibrant.

Also, movement supports brain health and functioning in many ways by helping new neurons to grow and thrive (as neurogenesis means the synthesis of neurons). Every day, our brains produce thousands of neurons, especially in our hippocampal region. This area is involved in learning and memory.

Movement or any kind of physical activity, whether it is skilled or simple like ordinary exercises that improve circulation, gives the new cells a purpose that they can engage in instead of dying. Thus, movement or being physically active helps maintain brain structures, slow age-related mental health, and speed mental recovery if the brain is injured or inflamed. It increases the level of a substance known as brain-derived neurotrophic factor or BDNF which is involved in learning and memory.

I hope we have considered how physical activity and physical-mental wellness are correlated, as exercise boosts both body and mind cells, and makes them engaged, have a purpose, and stay away from helplessness and hopelessness thus severe illness then death.

My advice if you fail to find any physical activity that encourages you, is to attend any social charity activities like feeding poor people, visiting or helping ill or disabled people, or even attending religious practices or gatherings.

As an interesting finding, religiousness (that is, people's personal involvement in religion) is associated with lower anxiety and depression, better physical health and longer life. Some religions promote a healthy lifestyle, such as avoiding smoking or alcohol, motivating people to help others, as well as social contact and support religious gatherings can provide.

Also, you can participate in educating others or bringing joy to people or children in restricted or sad conditions. Thereby enhancing your self-satisfaction as you embrace contentment by doing something valuable or helpful other than enhancing social communication which also boosts your immune system tremendously.

Research revealed that finding valuable meaning in your life and enhancing your purpose in life is a number one buffer to stress and the major booster of your immunity.

PART 5: PERSONALITY HARDINESS AND STRESS.

FOCUS
- How personality hardiness or toughness has a major effect on stress control.
- What is meant by personality strengths and how does it affect health?
- The positive, beneficial consequences of having personality strengths.
- How does the five-factor model of personality relate to health?

How personality hardiness or toughness has a major effect on stress control.

There are some personality factors that make the individual more able to withstand high levels of stressful experiences without becoming emotionally distressed or physically ill and other aspects of personality which make them more susceptible to these problems.

Early in the development of the field of health psychology, researchers Suzanne Kobasa and Salvatore Maddi suggested that individual differences in personal control provide only part of the reason why some people who are under stress get sick, whereas others do not.

They proposed that a broader array of personality traits called **hardiness** differentiates people who do and do not get sick under stress. The attitudes of hardiness are control, commitment and challenge. **Control** refers to people's belief that they can influence events in their lives. **Commitment** is a sense of personal control which means that people's sense of purpose is involved in the events, activities, and purpose in their lives.

For example, people with a strong sense of commitment tend to look forward to starting each day's project and enjoy getting close to people.

Challenge refers to the tendency to view changes as incentives or opportunities for growth rather than threats to security. The concept of hardiness has been highly influential, although more recent studies have found conflicting results and some evidence indicates that tests used to measure hardiness may simply be measuring the tendency to experience negative effects, such as the tendency to be anxious, depressed or hostile.

Nonetheless, the basic idea that some personality traits make the individual resilient has continued to be a major focus in the field and research supports this general hypothesis.

A personality concept that is similar to hardiness, is the **sense of coherence**. This trait involves the tendency of people to see their world as comprehensible, manageable and meaningful. People's sense of coherence has been linked to reduced levels of stress and illness symptoms. A related personality trait is the **sense of mastery**, which refers to people's general belief that they are able to deal effectively with the events of life rather than being subjected to forces beyond their control.

This trait is very similar to the belief in personal control, or a general sense of self-efficacy as described previously.

Optimism is the point of view that good things are likely to happen. Optimists tend to experience life's difficulties with less distress than pessimists do. They also tend to have better health habits, better mental and physical health and a faster recovery when they become ill than pessimists.

Finally, **resilience** refers to high levels of three interrelated positive components of personality: self-esteem, personal control and optimism. Resilient people appraise negative events as less stressful; they bounce back from their adversities and recover their strength and spirit.

Resilient children develop into competent, well-adjusted individuals even when growing up under extremely difficult conditions. Resilient people seem to make use of positive emotions and find meaning in the experience. Although such resilience was once considered rare, it now appears that probably most adults move on with their lives and do not suffer serious depression after a trauma, such as the loss of a close person like a parent or a friend or a partner.

Why are some people resilient and others not?

Part of the answer may lie in genetic endowments. Resilient people may have inherited traits, such as relatively easy temperaments, that enable them to cope better with stress and turmoil. Another part lies in their experiences. Resilient people who overcome a history of stressful events often have compensating experiences and circumstances in their lives, such as special talents or interests that absorb them and give them confidence and close relationships with friends or relatives.

The concepts of hardiness, resilience, optimism, mastery and coherence have a great deal in common and research scales used to measure these traits may be overlapping what is called **personality strengths.**

What is meant by personality strengths and how does it affect health?

Given the personality assets or strengths reflected in a sense of coherence, mastery and optimism, as a result, the spiralling process that can lead from stress to illness should not take hold. Studies have generally supported the prediction that these traits should be associated with lower risks of physical illness.

A meta-analysis of several studies of a variety of health conditions found that as expected optimism is associated with a reduced risk of developing physical illness and with a more positive outcome of illness among individuals who are already suffering from a disease.

Prospective studies have shown that optimistic people are at a lower risk of life-threatening conditions, such as heart disease. They have also found that people who have a strong sense of coherence had far lower mortality rates from cardiovascular disease and cancer over a six-year period than people low on this trait, and a sense of mastery has similar beneficial effects over time.

The positive, beneficial consequences of having personality strengths.

The personality strengths seem to correlate consistently with emotionally stability, the opposite of neuroticism and its components, such as anxiety or depressive symptoms and irritability which predict earlier death and several other negative health outcomes.

However, positive aspects of personality generally predict good future health even when the possibly overlapping effects of emotional stability versus neuroticism are taken into account.

Measures of personality strengths like optimism, mastery and sense of coherence also correlate with others in the five-factor model trait, especially, extroversion, conscientiousness, and openness. These traits also predict longevity and other health outcomes.

How does the five-factor model of personality relate to health?

Before knowing the answer to this question, here are some examples of each personality trait or dimension and its specific characteristics:

Neuroticism versus emotionally stable

A tendency to experience negative emotions, for example, anxiety, tension, sadness, irritability, feeling vulnerable, and unable to cope with stress versus calmness, even-tempered, relaxed, and able to deal with stressful situations without undue stress.

Extroversion versus introversion

Outgoing, gregarious, cheerful, talkative, interpersonal style, excitement seeking, assertiveness, and a tendency to experience positive emotions versus a reserved enjoyment of and even preference for solitude and quite subdued.

Openness versus closed mindset

Drawn to new experiences, open mindset, intellectual curiosity, readiness to examine and reconsider values and beliefs, try new things, "in touch" with feelings and aesthetic experience versus a dislike of change, rigid, dogmatic, narrow-minded.

Agreeableness versus antagonism

Altruistic, high empathy and concern for others, warm, forgiving, trusting, helpful, cooperative, and straightforward versus cold-hearted, cynical, guarded, disingenuous, mistrusting, argumentative, competitive, arrogant, and critical.

Conscientiousness versus unreliability

High self-control, organised, purposefulness, the self-image of being capable, prepared, competent, preference for order, dependable, printable, deliberate, self-disciplined, and achievement striving versus unorganised, low ambition, lackadaisical, and procrastinatory.

Now, the answer to how personality traits impact health significantly become vibrant, as mentioned, the assessment of stress and our response to it depend on our cognitive assessment that is interacted with our personality traits. Positive traits included in the five-factor model are also linked to one of the best-known **physiological modifiers** of stress.

People with such traits, experience less exposure to stressors at work and in relationships with less physiological reactivity, better recovery and better restoration, as reflected in better sleep and lower levels of physiological stress responses during sleep. In contrast, negative personality traits are linked to poor health. People with negative traits consistently experience greater exposure to stressors, greater reactivity, poorer recovery and poorer restoration.

PART 6: BEHAVIOUR AND EMOTIONAL STYLE AND STRESS.

FOCUS
- What is the Type A or B behavioural and emotional style?
- The impact of behavioural patterns on health.
- Type A behaviour and coronary heart disease (CHD).
- Hostility, anger and other negative emotions and CHD.

<u>What is the Type A or B behavioural and emotional style?</u>

Serendipity led to the discovery of the Type A behaviour pattern. Cardiologists Meyer Friedman and Ray Rosenman were studying the diets of male heart disease patients and their wives when one of the wives exclaimed:

"If you really want to know what is giving our husbands heart attacks, I will tell you. It is stress, the stress they receive in their work, that is what's doing it."

These researchers began to study this possibility and noticed that heart patients were more likely than non-patients to display a pattern of behaviour we now refer to as Type A.

Type A behavioural pattern characteristics

The Type A behaviour pattern consists of four characteristics:

Competitive achievement orientation

Type A individuals strive toward goals with a sense of being in competition with others and not feeling a sense of joy in their efforts or accomplishments.

Time urgency

Type A people seem to be in a constant struggle against the clock. Often, they quickly become impatient with delays and unproductive time. They schedule commitments too highly and try to do more than one thing at a time, such as reading while eating or watching TV.

Anger or hostility

Type A individuals tend to be easily aroused to anger or hostility which they may or may not express overtly.

Vigorous vocal style

Type A people speak loudly, rapidly and emphatically, often "taking over" and generally controlling the conversation.

Type B behavioural pattern characteristics

In contrast, the Type B behaviour pattern consists of low levels of competitiveness, time urgency and hostility.

People with the Type B pattern tend to be more easy-going and philosophical about life, and they are more likely to stop and smell the roses. In conversations, their speech is slower, and softer and reflects a more relaxed give and take.

The impact of behavioural patterns on health

Individuals who exhibit Type A behaviour patterns react differently to stressors from those with Type B patterns. Type A individuals respond more quickly and strongly to stressors, often interpreting them as threats to their personal control.

Type A individuals also often choose more demanding or pressured activities at work and in their leisure time and they often evoke angry and competitive behaviour from others. Hence, they have greater exposure to stressors too.

As I mentioned earlier, the response to a stressor or strain includes a physiological component called **reactivity**, such as an increase in blood pressure, catecholamines or cortisol levels compared to baseline levels. Type A's often show greater reactivity to stressors than Type B's, especially during situations involving competition, debates and arguments or other stressful social interactions.

People with Type A behaviour are at a greater risk than people with Type B behaviour of becoming sick with any variety of illnesses, such as asthma and indigestion.

Type A behaviour and coronary heart disease (CHD)

The narrowing of the coronary arteries that supply blood to heart muscles is called **atherosclerosis** and causes several manifestations of CHD. **Angina** is chest pain that occurs when the supply of oxygen carried by the blood to the heart muscle is not sufficient to meet the muscle's demand. When the demand exceeds the supply available through the narrowed coronary arteries and the heart is not getting enough oxygen, the heart muscle becomes **ischemic**. If the blood supply is blocked severely enough and for a long period of time, the ischemic portion of the heart muscle dies. This is called **myocardial infarction**, or what is commonly called a **heart attack**. A severely ischemic heart sometimes develops a lethal disturbance in rhythm, causing it to stop pumping blood throughout the body.

This is the usual cause of sudden cardiac death, where the patient dies within a few minutes or hours of first noticing symptoms. Dozens of studies have been done to assess the link between Type A behaviour and CHD, particularly anger or hostility which seems to be Type A's deadly emotions.

Hostility, anger and other negative emotions and CHD

People who are chronically hostile have an increased risk of developing CHD. The following study supports this idea.

Researchers examined the records of 225 doctors who had taken a psychological test that included a scale for hostility while they were in medical school 25 years earlier. For the doctors with high scores on the hostile scale, the rates of both CHD and overall mortality during the intervening years were several times higher than for those with low hostility scores.

The researchers measured hostility with a widely used test, the Cook Medley Hostility Scale, which has 50 true or false questions. This scale measures anger as well as, cynicism, suspiciousness and other negative traits.

In pursuing anger and hostility as the toxic element with the Type A pattern, a wide variety of self-reports and behavioural measures of these traits have been used.

A meta-analysis of the many studies on this topic found that anger and hostility are associated with an increased risk of CHD in initially healthy individuals. Furthermore, among people who already have CHD, anger and hostility are associated with an increased risk of poor medical outcomes such as additional heart attacks, or death from CHD.

Here again, the four stress processes of exposure, reactivity, recovery and restoration seem important. Angry and hostile people experience more conflict with others at home and work indicating greater exposure. The suspicious and mistrusting style of hostile people is likely to make them cold and argumentative during interactions with others. Sometimes, even with friends and family members.

The resulting conflict and reduced social support may, in turn, contribute to the maintenance or even worsening of their hostile behaviour toward others in a vicious cycle of self-fulfilling prophecy. Further, in difficult interpersonal situations in general, at work and with family members in particular, they show greater physiological reactivity or strain.

Moreover, unlike non-hostile people, hostile people do not respond to social support with reduced physiological reactivity during stressful situations, perhaps because they are too distrustful or worry that support providers will evaluate them negatively.

After a stressful situation, hostile people show delayed or incomplete recovery of their physiological stress responses, perhaps because they are more likely to brood or ruminate over upsetting events. Also, their sleep quality is more likely to suffer during stressful periods.

Combined, these stress processes can produce a lot of wear and tear on the cardiovascular system which in turn contributes to coronary atherosclerosis and the development of other indications of CHD. However, these stress processes might not be the only link between anger or hostility and CHD.

Anger and hostility are related to several unhealthy conditions and behaviours, such as heavy drinking, obesity and cigarette smoking that put people at risk of CHD. Although anger and hostility are generally associated with CHD even when these health behaviours and conditions are taken into account, some evidence suggests that they are at least part of the link between these personality traits and health.

Other negative heart health consequences of Type A pattern

Anger might not be the only unhealthy Type A behaviour, **social dominance**, and the tendency to exert

65

power, control or influence over other people are also associated with coronary atherosclerosis. In addition, this personality trait is associated with a greater physiological strain during challenging interpersonal tasks and situations like arguments and debates and efforts to influence others also evoke a larger increase in blood pressure and stress hormones. Type A behaviour especially the anger or hostility component is associated with increased stress and cardiovascular diseases.

So, we have seen how personality strengths and aspects of behaviour patterns are factors that can modify the impact of stress on health. This reveals the role of emotional style thus behaviour in either preventing or developing stress thus endangering heart health. Next, we will see how stress or negative coping (negative mindset) impairs health and causes major illnesses.

PART 7: STRESS AND ITS CRITICAL BODILY PHYSIOLOGICAL CHANGES.

FOCUS

- Stress negatively impacts different body systems.
- Stress affects cardiovascular system reactivity thus heart disease.
- Stress or negative feelings are a major factor in developing hypertension and CHD.

<u>Stress negatively impacts different body systems</u>

Connections have been found between illness and the degree of reactivity people show in their **cardiovascular**, **endocrine** and **immune systems** when stressed. We will discuss this in detail.

Under stress, the central nervous system (CNS) is in charge of your fight or flight response. In your brain, the hypothalamus gets the ball rolling, telling your adrenal glands to release the stress hormones adrenaline and cortisol. These hormones increase your heartbeat and send blood rushing to the areas that need it the most in an emergency, such as your muscles, heart, and other important organs.

When the perceived fear is gone, the hypothalamus should tell all systems to go back to normal. If the CNS fails to return to normal, or if the stressor doesn't go away, the response will continue. This is aligned with the aforementioned concept of allostatic load in which the strain is involved in reacting repeatedly to intense stressors producing wear and tear on body systems that accumulate over time and lead to illness.

A study found that for elderly individuals whose allostatic loads increased or decreased across a three-year period, those with increased loads had higher mortality rates during the next four years.

Chronic stress is also a major factor in developing negative behaviours such as overeating or not eating enough, alcohol or drug abuse, and social withdrawal.

Respiratory and cardiovascular systems

Stress hormones affect your respiratory and cardiovascular systems. During the stress response, you breathe faster in an effort to quickly distribute oxygen-rich blood to your body. If you already have a breathing problem like asthma or emphysema, stress can make it even harder to breathe.

Under stress, your heart also pumps faster. Stress hormones cause your blood vessels to constrict and divert more oxygen to your muscles so you'll have more strength to take action. But this also raises your blood pressure. As a result, frequent or chronic stress will make your heart work too hard for too long. When your blood pressure rises, so does your risk of having a stroke or heart attack.

Digestive system

Under stress, your liver produces extra blood sugar (glucose) to give you a boost of energy. If you're under chronic stress, your body may not be able to keep up with this extra glucose surge. Chronic stress may increase your risk of developing Type 2 diabetes.

The rush of hormones, rapid breathing, and increased heart rate can also upset your digestive system. You're more likely to have heartburn or acid reflux thanks to an increase in stomach acid. Stress does not cause ulcers (a bacterium called *H. pylori* often does), but it can increase your risk for them and cause existing ulcers to act up.

Stress can also affect the way food moves through your body, leading to diarrhoea or constipation. You might also experience nausea, vomiting, or a stomach ache.

Muscular system

Your muscles tense up to protect themselves from injury when you are stressed. They tend to release again once you relax, but if you are constantly under stress, your muscles may not get the chance to relax. Tight muscles cause headaches, back and shoulder pain, and body aches. Over time, this can set off an unhealthy cycle as you stop exercising and turn to pain medication for relief.

Sexuality and reproductive system

Stress is exhausting for both the body and mind. It is not unusual to lose your desire when you're under constant stress.

While short-term stress may cause men to produce more of the male hormone testosterone, this effect doesn't last. If stress continues for a long time, a man's testosterone levels can begin to drop. This can interfere with sperm production and cause erectile dysfunction or impotence. Chronic stress may also increase the risk of infection for male reproductive organs like the prostate and testes.

For women, stress can affect the menstrual cycle. It can lead to irregular, heavier, or more painful periods. Chronic stress can also magnify the physical symptoms of menopause.

Stress affects cardiovascular system reactivity thus heart disease

Cardiovascular reactivity refers to the physiological changes that occur in the heart, blood vessels and blood in response to stressors. Before middle age, people's degree of cardiovascular reactivity is generally stable, showing little change when rested, with the same stressors years later. In later years, cardiovascular reactivity increases with age, which corresponds to an increased risk of cardiovascular illness.

Research has discovered links between high cardiovascular reactivity and the development of CHD, hypertension, and stroke. Stress is a major contributor to heart disease.

Research revealed that high levels of job stress are associated with high blood pressure and abnormally enlarged hearts, and people's laboratory reactivity to stress in early adulthood correlated with their later development of high blood pressure and atherosclerosis. The blood pressure reactivity that people display in laboratory tests appears to reflect their reactivity in daily life.

A meta-analysis found that greater cardiovascular reactivity and poor cardiovascular recovery after stressors were associated with a greater risk of cardiovascular disease, including high blood pressure, diagnosed hypertension and atherosclerosis. Stress produces several cardiovascular changes that relate to the development of CHD.

For example, the blood of people who are under stress contains high concentrations of activated platelets and clotting factors that thicken the blood which can contribute to a heart attack. Stress also produces unfavourable levels of cholesterol and inflammatory substances circulating in the blood.

These changes in blood composition promote atherosclerosis within artery walls. These changes narrow and stiffen the arteries thereby increasing blood pressure and the risk of a heart attack or stroke.

Researchers Stephen Manuck et al (1975) have demonstrated this link between stress and atherosclerosis in research with monkeys.

In one study over many months, some of the subjects were relocated periodically to different living groups. This required stressful adjustments among the animals as they sought to re-establish the social hierarchies these animals naturally form, especially for higher ranking or dominant animals to retain their status. The remaining subjects stayed in stable living groups.

The stressed monkeys who tended to hold dominant status in their living groups developed greater atherosclerosis than the dominant animals in the low-stress condition, and greater than the lower-ranking or subordinate monkeys in their living condition. These effects were prevented when the animals were given a drug that blocked the sympathetic nervous system excitation of the heart muscle, strongly implicating the role of chronic or recurring activation of the fight or flight response in the development of atherosclerosis.

Similar effects of experimentally manipulated stressful living conditions on atherosclerosis have been demonstrated in rabbits.

Although, human stress and cardiovascular disease probably differ somewhat from what occurs in these animals. The ability to perform true experiments in which chronic stress is manipulated over long periods of time provides important converging evidence to the findings of observational studies of human stress and cardiovascular disease.

Recent research suggests that it is not just the **excitatory effects** of the sympathetic nervous system on the cardiovascular system that contribute to cardiovascular disease. If this activating system functions like an accelerator in activating stress responses, the **parasympathetic nervous system** brakes on such reactivity which is also important.

The functioning of this stress-dampening system can be measured through increases and decreases in heart rate that are due to respiration. Changes in the activity of the parasympathetic nervous system cause the heart rate to slow down when we breathe in. The magnitude of this change in heart rate, sometimes called **vagal tone** because it is caused by the activity of the vagus nerve, is a good indicator of the strength of an individual's parasympathetic stress-dampening system.

Importantly, a higher vagal tone is associated with a lower risk of cardiovascular disease, that is, parasympathetic brakes on stress are protective. This means that stress impacts on our bodies can be controlled by the parasympathetic nervous system and can be healthier and stronger according to one's mindset positivity, thus their behaviour type.

People can control stress's negative impact and assess its wide effect on body functioning by using their parasympathetic nervous system as a brake to the rushed, powerful body response to stress.

Bodily response to stress or negative mindset contributes to cardiovascular disorder development

The condition of having high blood pressure consistently over several weeks or more is a major risk factor for CHD, stroke and kidney disease. Recent statistics of the past 20 years worldwide revealed a significant increase in hypertension.

For example, in the USA, nearly 30% of adults are classified as hypertensive, having blood pressure at or above 140 systolic over 90 diastolic. By comparison, the hypertension rates elsewhere are as follows: Australia, 21% to 32%; Canada, 20%; Europe, 44%; across several nations worldwide, 26%.

Note: Because a lesser elevation in blood pressure is now known to increase the risk substantially, current guidelines designate less than 120/80 as normal or conveying little risk. Prevalence rates for hypertension increase in adulthood particularly after 40 years of age.

Why do people develop hypertension?

Some cases of hypertension are caused by or are secondary to disorders of other body systems or organs such as the kidneys or endocrine system. Secondary hypertension can usually be cured by medical procedures but, the vast majority over 90% of hypertension cases are classified as primary or essential hypertension in which the causes of high blood pressure are unknown.

To say the causes of essential hypertension are unknown is somewhat misleading. In cases of essential hypertension, doctors are unable to identify any biomedical causes, such as infectious agents or organ damage. But many risk factors are associated with the development of hypertension. And there is evidence implicating the following as some of the risk factors for hypertension:

- Obesity
- Dietary elements such as high salt, fats and cholesterol
- Excessive alcohol use
- Physical inactivity
- Family history of hypertension
- Psychological factors such as chronic stress anger and anxiety

Stress or negative feelings is a major factor in developing hypertension and CHD

People's occupations provide sources of stress that can have an impact on their blood pressure.

Researchers Sidney Cobb and Robert Rose (1973) compared the medical records of thousands of men employed as air traffic controllers or as second-class airmen separating the data by different age groups since blood pressure increases with age. Comparisons for each group revealed rates of hypertension among air traffic controllers that were several times higher than for the airmen. The researchers also compared the records of air traffic controllers who experienced high and low levels of stress as measured by the traffic density at the air stations where they worked.

The study depicts that for each age group, prevalence rates of hypertension were higher for air traffic controllers working at high-stress locations than for those at low-stress sites.

Other research showed that aspects of the social environment such as crowding and aggression are also linked to stress and hypertension. Experiments with animals have shown that living in crowded and aggressive conditions induces chronic hypertension.

Research with humans compared people living in crowded and uncrowded neighbourhoods to see if these living conditions influence blood pressure. The people from the two types of neighbourhoods were similar in important characteristics such as age, gender, and family income. While working on a stressful cognitive task, the subjects showed a greater increase in heart rate and systolic and diastolic pressure if they lived in a crowded neighbourhood.

Other research has found that psychological stress and high cardiovascular reactivity stress may be a risk factor for or even a cause of hypertension. Taken together, the evidence suggests that chronic stress plays a role in the development of hypertension.

Negative feelings stemmed from a negative mindset and hypertension

Studies on pessimism, anger and hostility have revealed important links to the development of hypertension. We will consider three:

First, blood pressure is higher in pessimistic than optimistic individuals.

Second, people who are hypertensive are more likely to be chronically hostile and resentful than normotensive people (those with normal blood pressure). Anger is also associated with higher night-time blood pressure.

Third, resting blood pressure is higher among individuals who ruminate or dwell on events that provoke anger than among people who do not ruminate.

Interestingly, the effects of stress on blood pressure can complicate the medical diagnosis of hypertension. Some people become anxious when medical professionals measure their blood pressure, producing an elevated reading that actually is not responsive to their usual blood pressure levels, leading to a false diagnosis of hypertension. If undetected this **white-coat hypertension** can lead to unnecessary medical treatment.

Psychological stress (negative emotions) and CHD

Epidemiologists have studied the distribution and frequency of CHD over many decades in many different cultures. The data they have collected suggests that CHD is to some extent, a disease of modernised societies, meaning, the incidence rate of heart disease is higher in technologically advanced countries than in other nations. This may be due to people in advanced societies living long enough to become patients of CHD, which afflicts mainly older individuals. There are also other factors, such as obesity and low levels of physical activity.

The major factor is due to the psychosocial stressors of advanced societies that may be more conducive to the development of heart disease. People in less advanced countries may have more social support to protect themselves from the effects of stress and perceive less reason for anger and hostility which we have already seen can increase the risk of CHD.

Research assures the link between stress (negative mindset), thinking or feeling and CHD

Studies revealed that job stress, conflict in close relationships, post-traumatic stress disorder and stress-related personality factors like anger and pessimism predict the development of CHD. Associations between stress and myocardial infarction or death from CHD could occur across various phases of the disease.

Stress could contribute to the initiation and progression of atherosclerosis, even years before the first symptoms and other outwards indications of CHD occurred. Later, in the presence of advanced atherosclerosis, stress contributes to the occurrence of ischemia, myocardial infarction or disturbances in the rhythm of the heart that reveal clinically apparent CHD. Still, later, stress could contribute to impaired health outcomes for people with established CHD, such as additional heart attacks or coronary death. Research has supported each of these possibilities.

For example, anger is associated with stiffness in arteries that indicate very early signs of atherosclerosis.

Research has also found higher levels of atherosclerosis in the arteries of African-American women who perceived high levels of stress and experienced unfair treatment and racial discrimination in their lives than those who did not. Also, having experiences of high demand and low control in dealing with daily stressors is associated with a greater progression of atherosclerosis over time.

Later in the development of CHD, a variety of stressful and negative emotions, such as episodes of anger, can participate in a heart attack in people with advanced atherosclerosis. Finally, anger, depression and stressful aspects of neighbourhoods have all been found to predict poor medical outcomes, including recurring heart attacks and death in CHD patients.

PART 8: STRESS AND NEGATIVE HEALTH IMPACT AND CANCER.

FOCUS

- Stress (negative mindset) produces other physiological changes that contribute to the development of cancer.
- The immune system and its organs and functions.
- Stress or negative emotions and the immune system.
- Other health hazards as a result of stress or a negative mindset.
- Final brief guidelines to enhance positive mindset and thus health status.

Stress (negative mindset) produces other physiological changes that contribute to the development of cancer

This idea has a long history since the physician Galen predicted it in Rome during the second century A.D. He believed that individuals who were sad and depressed or melancholy were more likely to develop cancer than those who were happy, confident and vigorous. Similar ideas have appeared in the writings of doctors in later eras.

Cancer is the term that refers to a broad class of diseases in which cells multiply and grow in an unrestrained manner. Therefore, cancer does not refer to a single illness but to dozens of disease forms that share this characteristic. It includes, for instance, leukaemia, in which the bone marrow produces excessive numbers of white blood cells and carcinoma in which tumours form in the tissue of the skin and internal organ linings. Some cancers take longer to develop or follow more irregular courses in their development than others do.

Early evidence linking stress and cancer came from research using retrospective methods. This research generally had cancer patients fill out a life event questionnaire to assess the stress they experienced during the year or so preceding the diagnosis.
Although some studies found that the appearance of cancer was associated with self-reported high levels of prior stress, others did not. However, the following problems with retrospective methods cloud the interpretation of the results of these studies:

1. The cancer diagnoses were typically made years after the disease process started.

2. The patients' cancers were probably present prior to and during the year for which they reported high levels of stress.

3. The patients' perception or recollection of prior stress may have been distorted by their knowledge that they have cancer.

More recent and better-diagnosed research, using prospective and longitudinal approaches, also has inconsistent results. But, a meta-analysis of a large number of available studies indicated that stress-related psychosocial factors predicted the initial occurrence of cancer, as well as the medical course of the disease including survival and death from cancer.

The effects of stress on cancer are probably influenced by many factors. If stress plays a causal role in cancer development or progression, this may be due to it impairing the immune system's ability to combat the disease by increasing behavioural risk factors such as smoking. As in the case of CHD, cancer progresses in a complex manner.

Cancer progression eventually involves the recruitment of a blood supply to permit the growth of the tumour beyond the early stages called **angiogenesis**. Furthermore, cancer can spread beyond the tissue where it originally occurred, a process called **metastasis**.

Recently, research has begun to identify ways in which physiological stress responses can influence angiogenesis as well as the health behaviour and immune system mechanisms traditionally thought to link stress and cancer. Let us see this in detail, firstly looking at the immune system.

The immune system and its organs and functions

The immune system fights to defend the body against "foreign invaders" such as bacteria and viruses. It is known, that this system is highly sensitive to invasions by foreign matter and is able to distinguish between self or normal body constituents (friend) and non-self (foe).

What are antigens?

When the body recognises something as non-self, the immune system mobilises the body's resources and attacks. Any substance that can trigger an immune response is called an antigen as bacteria and viruses are recognized by the tallest aspects of their protein coats and DNA. The immune system also tends to recognise tissues of an organ transplant as non-self and treats them as an antigen. This is what doctors mean when they say that the body has rejected a transplant.

There are two basic ways to encourage transplant acceptance. The first is to select the transplant carefully so that the tissues of the donor and the recipient are closely matched. "The closer the genetic relationship between two people, the better the match is likely to be. Identical twins provide the best match, of course."

The second approach uses drugs to suppress parts of the immune system, so it will not mobilise and reject the organ. "A drawback to this approach is that suppressing immune function can leave the patient susceptible to disease."

For many people, the immune system amounts to an attack against normally harmless substances, such as pollen, tree mould, poison ivy, animal dander and particular foods. These people suffer from allergies, the specific substances that trigger their allergic reactions, such as sneezing and skin rashes are called allergens.

Most people with allergies react to some but not all of the known allergens, someone with hay fever may not be allergic to poison ivy, for instance. Being allergic is partly determined by heredity. Some allergies can be reduced by administering regular small doses of the allergen usually by injection.

The organs of the immune system are located throughout the body. These organs are generally referred to as lymphatic or lymphoid organs because they have a primary role in the development and the deployment of **lymphocytes**, specific white blood cells, that are the key functionaries or soldiers in our body's defence against invasion by foreign matter. The main lymphatic organs include the bone marrow, thymus, lymph nodes and vessels and spleen.

Lymphocytes originate in the bone marrow, the soft tissue in the core of all bones in the body, some of these cells migrate to one of two organs where they mature. One of these organs is the thymus, which is an endocrine gland that lies in the chest. The other organ is not known for certain but, it is thought to have the same function in maturating human lymphocytes that a structure called the bursa has in birds. Most of this processing of lymphocytes occurs before birth and in infancy.

The function of lymph nodes

The lymph nodes are bean-shaped masses of spongy tissue that are distributed throughout the body (large clusters of them are found in the neck, armpits, abdomen, and groin). Each lymph node contains filters that capture antigens and compartments that provide a home base for lymphocytes and other white blood cells. A network of lymph vessels that contains a clear fluid called lymph, connects the lymph nodes. These vessels ultimately empty into the bloodstream.

Although the lymph nodes and vessels play an important role in cleansing body cells of antigens, they can become a liability in some forms of cancer either by becoming infected with cancer or by distributing cancer cells to other parts of the body through the lymph and blood.

Lymphocytes and antigens that enter the blood are carried to the spleen, an organ in the upper left side of a person's abdomen. The spleen functions like an enormous lymph node except that blood rather than lymph travels through it. It filters out antigens and serves as a home base for white blood cells. It also removes ineffective or worn-out red blood cells from the body.

White blood cells play a key role in the immune system, they serve as soldiers in our counter-attack, against invading substances in the body. There are two types of white blood cells: lymphocytes as we have seen are one type; **phagocytes** are the other. Phagocytes are scavengers that patrol the body and engulf and ingest antigens. They are not choosy. They will eat anything suspicious that they find in the bloodstream, tissues or lymphatic system.

In the lungs, for instance, they consume particles of dust and other pollutants, that enter with each breath. They can clean lungs that have been blackened with the contaminants of cigarette smoke, provided that the smoking stops. Too much smoking over a long time destroys phagocytes faster than they can be replenished.

There are two main types of phagocytes: **macrophages** become attached to tissue and remain there and **neutrophils** circulate in the blood. The fact that phagocytes are not choosy means that they are involved in nonspecific immunity, they respond to any kind of antigen.

Lymphocytes react in a more discriminating way, being tailored for attacks against specific antigens, in addition to the process of nonspecific immunity. There are two types of specific immune processes: cell-mediated immunity and antibody-mediated (or humoral) immunity.

Let us examine these two specific immune responses and how they interrelate.

Cell-mediated immunity operates at the level of the cells. The soldiers in the process are lymphocytes called **T cells**, the name of these white cells reflects their having matured in the thymus.

T cells are divided into several groups, each with its own important function:

1. **Killer T cells** directly attack and destroy three main targets. Transplanted tissue that is recognised as foreign, cancerous cells, and cells of the body that have already been invaded by antigens such as viruses.

2. **Memory T cells** remember previous invaders. At the time of an initial infection, like with mumps, some of them are imprinted with information for recognising that specific kind of invader or the virus that causes mumps in the future. Thus, such cells and their offspring circulate in the blood for long periods of time and enable the body to defend against subsequent invasions more quickly.

3. **Delayed hypersensitivity T cells** have two functions. They are involved in delayed immune reactions, particularly in allergies, for instance, poison ivy, in which tissue becomes inflamed. They also produce protein

substances called **lymphokines** that stimulate other T cells to grow, reproduce and attack an invader.

4. **Helper T cells** (also called CD4 cells) receive reports of invasions from other white blood cells that patrol the body. They rush to the spleen and lymph nodes and stimulate lymphocytes to reproduce and attack. The lymphocytes they stimulate are from both the cell-mediated and the antibody-mediated immunity processes.

5. **Suppressor T cells** operate in slowing down or stopping cell-mediated and antibody-mediated immunity processes as an infection diminishes or is conquered.

Suppressor and helper T cells serve to regulate cell-mediated and antibody-mediated immune processes.

Antibody-mediated immunity attacks bacteria, fungi, protozoa and viruses while they are still in the bodily fluids and before they have invaded body cells. Unlike the cell-mediated process of attacking infected cells of the body, the antibody-mediated approach focuses on the antigens directly. The soldiers in this approach are lymphocytes called **B cells**, they give rise to plasma cells that produce antibodies. This process is often induced by helper T cells, or inherited by suppressor T cells.

Antibodies are protein molecules called immunoglobulin (Ig), that attach to the surface of invaders and accomplish three results.

Firstly, they slow down the invader making it an easier and more attractive target for phagocytes to destroy.

Secondly, they recruit other protein substances that puncture the membrane of an invading microorganism causing it to burst.

Thirdly, they find new invaders and form memory B cells that operate in the future like T cells, thus, antibodies are like sophisticated weapons in immune system wars.

Research has identified five classes of them (IgD, IgM, IgA, IgD, and IgE) each with a special function and territory in the body.

For example, IgA guards the entrance of organs in fluids, such as saliva, tears and secretions in the respiratory tract.

Stress or negative emotions and the immune system

People's emotions, both positive and negative, are the result of mindset and play a critical role in the balance and strength of immune functions. Research has shown that pessimism, depression, and stress from major and minor events are related to impaired immune function.

For example, the researchers compared the immune variables of caregiver spouses of Alzheimer's disease patients with matched control subjects and found that caregivers had a lower immune function and reported more days of illness over the course of about a year.

Positive emotions also affect immune function, giving it a boost, as the result of the study by Arthur Stone et al revealed. In the study, adult men kept daily logs of positive and negative events and gave saliva samples for analyses of antibody content. Negative events were associated with reduced antibodies only for the day the event occurred, but positive events enhanced antibody content for the day of occurrence and the next two days.

When people react to short-term, minor events like doing difficult maths problems under time pressure, changes in the number and activity of immune cells occur for fairly short periods (minutes or hours). The degree of change depends on which immune system components are measured, if the event's characteristics are long-lasting, and if intense interpersonal events seem to produce especially large immune reductions.

One key process of immune system inflammation is receiving increased attention because it is implicated in a wide variety of serious medical conditions. Stress can evoke increases in inflammatory substances in the blood as can chronic levels of negativity affect inflammation, which in turn can contribute to atherosclerosis, rheumatoid arthritis and other conditions, and seem to generally accelerate age-related diseases.

One confusing question in this area is the fact that one stress response, the release of cortisol, generally decreases inflammation. But emerging perspective agents suggest that under conditions of chronic stress, the immune system becomes less sensitive to the normal anti-inflammatory effects of cortisol, so that "inflammatory responses remain activated that can eventually damage health."

Research has confirmed the relationship between stress and illness. For instance, people who experience high levels of stress, contract more infectious diseases.

Is there a direct link between stress or a negative mindset and immune function? Yes, researchers from a variety of disciplines have researched to examine this link.

One study of first-year medical students, who were scheduled to take a series of highly stressful final examinations, assessed important variables in two sessions one month before the finals and one month after their last major exam.

In the first session, the researchers took a sample of blood from the students and had them fill out questionnaires that assessed their experiences of loneliness and stress during the past year. In the second session, only a blood sample was taken. Analyses of the samples revealed that killer T-cell activity was considerably lower in the second high-stress blood sample than in the first. It was also lower among students who scored high on the loneliness and stress questionnaires compared to those who scored low.

Another study analysed blood samples of married and separated or divorced women. This study found weaker immune function among married women who reported less marital satisfaction and among the separated or divorced women who refused to accept the separation or thought excessively about their ex-spouse compared to those who did not.

Studies by other researchers support these results finding, for example, weaker immune function during bereavement and after experiencing a natural disaster. Furthermore, people with a negative mindset engage in unhealthy behaviour which in turn contributes to a weakened immune system.

For example, unhealthy lifestyles such as, smoking cigarettes or being sedentary have been associated with impaired immune function.

Poor nutrition can also lead to a less-than-optimal immune function. Diets deficient in vitamins and minerals seem to diminish the production of lymphocytes and antibodies which adds more harm to the immune system functioning.

Other health hazards as a result of stress or a negative mindset

Stress as the cause of autoimmune disease

When your immune system functions optimally, it attacks foreign matter and protects the body. Sometimes, this process goes awry and the immune response is directed at parts of the body it should protect. Several disorders result from this condition, they are called **autoimmune diseases**.

One of these diseases is **rheumatoid arthritis** in which the immune response is directed against tissues and bones at the joints. This causes swelling and pain and can leave the bones pitted. In **rheumatic fever**, the muscles of the heart are the target, often leaving the heart valves permanently damaged.

Multiple sclerosis results when the immune system attacks the myelin sheath of neurons. Another autoimmune disease is **systemic lupus erythematosus** which affects various parts of the body, such as the skin and heart.

Evidence indicates that heredity and immune responses to prior infections play important roles in the development of autoimmune diseases. Stress or a negative mindset impairs the endocrine system reactivity and then the immune system reactivity thus leading to illnesses.

Part of the reactivity involves activation of the adrenal glands, both directly by sympathetic nervous system stimulation of these glands and by the hypothalamus-pituitary-adrenal axis, as described previously. In the process, the adrenal glands release hormones particularly catecholamine and corticosteroids during stress. The increased endocrine reactivity that people display in these tests appears to reflect their reactivity in daily life.

One way in which high levels of these hormones can lead to illness involves their effects on the cardiovascular system. Intense episodes of stress with high levels of hormones can lead to illness which in turn affects the cardiovascular system.

For example, an intense episode of stress with high levels of hormones can cause the heart to beat erratically and may even lead to sudden cardiac death.

In addition, chronically high levels of catecholamines and corticosteroids such as cortisol can contribute to the development and progression of atherosclerosis. As mentioned before, stress lowers endocrine reactivity. People with high levels of social support could be helped more than those with lower ones as social support exhibits lower endocrine reactivity.

Stress also seems to affect health through endocrine system pathways that involve fat stored in the abdominal cavity. **Metabolic syndrome** is a set of risk factors including, high levels of cholesterol and other blood fats, elevated blood pressure, high levels of insulin in the blood or impairments in the ability of insulin to facilitate transportation of glucose out of the bloodstream, and larger fat deposits in the abdomen.

Metabolic syndrome seems to be made worse by exposure to stressors and related physiological stress responses, especially heightened neuroendocrine activity. Metabolic syndrome also promotes chronic inflammation in the bloodstream and elsewhere, increasing the risk of cardiovascular diseases and other serious conditions like diabetes.

The impact of stress on the immune system reactivity

The release of catecholamines and corticosteroids during arousal affects health in another way. These stress responses alter the function of the immune system.

Brief stressors typically activate some components of the immune system, especially non-specific immunity, while suppressing specific immunity. **Chronic stressors** in contrast, more generally suppress both non-specific and specific immune functions. They also increase inflammation, an important process that disrupts immune function, when it occurs on a long-term basis. So, rather than a simple "up and down" effect of stress on this vital system, stress deregulates or disrupts it.

The effects of acute and chronic stress on the immune system can be measured in many ways, such as the extent to which the immune system cells multiply or proliferate in response to antigens, or the ability of such cells to destroy foreign microorganisms or viruses.

For example, an increase in cortisol and epinephrine is associated with decreased activity of T cells and B cells against antigens. This decrease in lymphocytic activity appears to be important in the development and progression of a variety of infectious diseases and cancer.

Those with high levels of killer T-cell activity have a better prognosis than those with low levels of activity.

Immune processes also protect the body against cancer that results from excessive exposure to harmful chemicals or physical agents called **carcinogens** which include radiation, tobacco smoke, and asbestos. Carcinogens can damage the DNA in the body's cells which may then develop into mutant cells and spread. Fortunately, people's exposure to carcinogens is generally at low levels and for a short period of time and most DNA changes probably do not lead to cancer.

When mutant cells develop, the immune system attacks them with killer T cells. Actually, the body begins to defend itself against cancer even before the cell mutates by using enzymes to destroy chemical carcinogens or to repair damaged DNA. But research has shown that high levels of stress reduce the production of these enzymes and the repair of damaged DNA. Thus, if stress disrupts the immune system, it can affect a great variety of health conditions from the common cold to herpes virus infections to cancer.

As shown, the psychological and biological systems are interrelated, as one system changes the other is often affected. This led researchers to form a new field of study called **psychoneuroimmunology**. This field focuses on the relationship between psychosocial processes and the activities of the nervous, endocrine and immune systems.

These systems form chemical messages in the form of neurotransmitters and hormones that increase or decrease immune function. And cells from the immune system produce chemicals, such as cytokines and ACTH, that feed the information back to the brain. The brain appears to serve as a control centre to maintain a balanced immune function since too little immune activity leaves the individual open to infection and too much activity may produce autoimmune disease.

Psychophysiological disorders

The word psychosomatic has a long history and was coined to refer to symptoms or illnesses that are caused or aggravated by psychological factors, mainly, emotional stress. Although many professionals and the general public still use this term, the concept has undergone some changes and now has a new name, **psychophysiological disorders**, which refers to physical symptoms or illnesses that result from the interplay of psychological and physiological processes.

This definition clearly used the following biopsychosocial perspective:

1. Digestive system diseases

Several psychophysiological disorders can affect the digestive system. **Ulcers** and **inflammatory bowel disease** are two illnesses that involve wounds in the digestive tract that may cause pain and bleeding. Ulcers are found in the stomach and the duodenum or upper section of the small intestine. Inflammatory bowel disease which includes ulcerative colitis and Crohn's disease can occur in the colon (large intestine), and the small intestine.

Another illness is **irritable bowel syndrome**, which produces abnormal pain, diarrhoea and constipation. Although these diseases afflict mainly adults, similar symptoms occur in childhood. Most ulcers are produced by a combination of gastric juices eroding the lining of the stomach and duodenum that has been weakened by bacterial infection. But stress plays a role, too.

In a classic study, a patient agreed to cooperate in a lengthy and detailed examination of gastric function. He was unique because many years earlier at the age of nine, he had a stomach operation that left an opening to the outside of the body.

This opening, which provided the only way he could feed himself was literally a window through which the inside of his stomach could be observed. When he was subjected to stressful situations, his stomach acid production greatly increased. When he was under emotional tension for several weeks, there was a pronounced reddening of the stomach lining.

Another study reported similar effects with a 15-month-old girl, who had a temporary stomach opening. Her highest level of acid secretion occurred when she was angry, the physical causes of inflammatory bowel disease and irritable bowel syndrome were not well known.

Stress is related to flare-ups of these illnesses, but its specific role is currently unclear.

2. Asthma

Asthma is a respiratory disorder in which inflammation, spasms and mucous obstruct the bronchial tubes and leads to difficulty in breathing, with wheezing or coughing. Asthma attacks appear to result from some combination of three factors: allergies, respiratory infections, and biopsychosocial arousal from stress or exercise, in most cases. The cause of an attack is largely physical but sometimes it may be largely psychosocial.

Professionals working with hospitalized children have noticed that the asthma symptoms of many children decrease shortly after admission to the hospital, but reappear when they return home. Are these children allergic to something in their houses? They tested that with asthmatic children who were allergic to house dust without the children knowing.

The researchers vacuumed the children's homes and then sprayed the collected dust from each house into their individual hospital rooms. The result: none of the children had respiratory difficulty when exposed to their home dust. This suggests that psychosocial factors have been implicated in the development of asthma, the occurrence of asthma attacks, and the inflammatory processes that worsen asthma attacks, including adversity during childhood and family patterns that involve stress and low social support. A meta-analysis of this research indicated that the association between stress-related psychosocial factors and asthma is bidirectional.

Stress and negative emotions can contribute to the development and worsening of asthma and having asthma can contribute to future stress and negative emotions.

3. Recurrent headaches

There are two types of the most common recurrent headaches: tension-type and migraine.

Tension-type, muscle contraction, seems to be caused by a combination of a central nervous system dysfunction and persistent contraction of the head and neck muscles. The pain it produces is a dull, and steady ache, often feeling like a tight band of pressure around the head. Recurrent tension-type headaches occur twice a week or more and may last for hours, days or weeks.

Migraines seem to result from the dilation of blood vessels surrounding the brain and dysfunction in the brain stream and trigeminal nerve that extends throughout the front half of the head. The pain, which often begins on the side of the head near the temple, is sharp and throbbing and lasts for hours or sometimes days. Sometimes, migraines begin with or follow an aura, a set of symptoms that signal an impending headache episode. These symptoms usually include sensory phenomena, such as seeing lines or shimmering in the visual fields. This may be accompanied by dizziness, nausea and vomiting.

What triggers headaches? They are often brought on by hormonal changes, missing a meal, sunlight, sleeping poorly, and consuming certain substances like alcohol or tobacco. Research has shown that stressors, particularly the hassles of everyday living are common triggers of migraines.

Thus, stress or a negative mindset seems to be one of the major causes that contribute to the production of such headaches.

4. Other disorders

Stress appears to be involved in triggering or aggravating episodes of illnesses such as rheumatoid arthritis, a chronic and very painful disease that produces inflammation and stiffness of the small joints like in the hands. It affects about 1% of the American population and its victims are primarily women. Stress seems to play a role in arthritis inflammation, pain and limitations in physical activity.

Another disorder called **dysmenorrhea** affects millions of women. It is characterised by painful menstruation that may be accompanied by nausea, headache and dizziness. A third stress-related problem involves skin disorders, such as **hives**, **eczema** and **psoriasis** in which the skin develops rashes or becomes dry and flakes or cracks. In many cases, specific allergies are identified as contributing to episodes of these skin problems.

We have seen that beliefs and mindset lead to action behaviours that then affect lifestyle type thus affecting one's body responses and health.

Final brief guidelines to enhance positive mindset and thus health status

Mortality from today's leading cause of death could be markedly reduced, if people adopted a few health behaviours and a simple healthy lifestyle like quitting smoking, avoiding or limiting alcohol, eating a healthy diet, and exercising regularly.

Thus, it is crucial for us to become fairly consistent with health practices to help ourselves engage easily in healthy behaviours and decisions at critical times. As such health-related behaviours that become well-established often become habitual, thus enhancing our wellness under any or all life events.

In order to adhere to such healthy practices, it is very essential to maintain a positive mental status and to control stress by learning to cope with it if it is out of our control. Coping is the process by which people try to manage the real or perceived discrepancy between the demands and the resources they appraise in stressful situations, as detailed in the first part of the book. So, we have to push ourselves towards rationality, motivate ourselves towards seeking our goals in a realistic and systematic way and keep rehearsing the positive outcomes of being committed to the right path.

Also, as known, coping with stress through transactions with the environment that do not necessarily lead to solutions to the problems causes stress. So, people can reduce the potential of stress in their lives and others' lives in several ways:

Firstly, we can increase the social support we give and receive by joining social, cultural and special interest groups.

Secondly, we can improve our own and others' sense of personal control and hardiness by taking responsibility for our roles and actions in life, learning, and never engaging in blaming others' thinking patterns as this is the trigger of a negative mindset and its detrimental consequences.

For example, we can reduce frustration and waste less time by organising our world better via wise-assertive time management, re-ordering our responsibilities realistically, focusing on our priorities and making a timeline for each without expecting perfection while being flexible if we failed or felt that things have gone out of our control.

Thirdly, by exercising and keeping fit – at least, being physically active we can reduce the experience of stress and the negative impact it has on our health.

Fourthly and most importantly, learn how to prepare for stressful events.

For example, a medical procedure is a really stressful event we can cope with by improving our behavioural, cognitive and informational control. So, we must consider its valuable outcome rather than the fear of its pain or risk and adhere to all the required health strategies to assure its success. This could never be achieved without a positive mindset that accepts, assesses rationally and acts wisely in any and every helpful way.

Also, there are many stress management methods that we must learn and consider to alleviate the impact of real stressors, such as:

1. Progressive muscle relaxation, systematic desensitization, biofeedback, modelling, and several approaches.

2. Cognitive therapy attempts to modify stress-producing and irrational thought patterns through the process of cognitive restructuring.

3. Stress inoculation training and problem-solving training are designed to teach people skills to alleviate stress and achieve personal goals.

4. Beneficial effects have been found for all of the behavioural and cognitive stress management methods, particularly, relaxation, massage, meditation and hypnosis have been shown to help reduce stress, too.

Be informed that stress management techniques can also reduce coronary risk, treating hypertension. Also, by modifying Type A behaviour via rational self-talk (see below) to confront each negative behaviour in order to feel peaceful and calm then acting positively, reverses or at least determines illness.

The following is an example of rational self-talk:

1. Preparation for provocation

This could be a rough situation, but I know how to deal with it. I can work out a plan to handle this. Easy does it. Remember, stick to the issues and don't take them personally. There won't be any need for an argument, I know what to do.

2. Impact and confrontation

As long as I keep my cool, I'm in control of the situation. I do not need to prove myself. Do not make more out of this than I have to. There is no point in getting frustrated. Think of what I have to do. Look for the positives and do not jump to conclusions.

3. Coping with Arousal

My muscles are getting tight. Relax and slow things down. Time to take a deep breath. Let's take the issue point by point. My anger is a signal of what I need to do. Time for problem-solving, maybe that person wants me to get angry or perhaps that situation provokes great anxiety but, I am going to deal with it constructively.

4. Subsequent Reflection

Unresolved conflict – forget about the aggravation. Thinking about it only makes me upset. Try to shake it off. Do not let it interfere with my job. Remember relaxation is a lot better than anger. Don't take it personally. It's probably not that big of a deal.

5. Conflict resolved

I handled that one pretty well. That's doing a good job. I could have gotten more upset than it was worth. I should not take it as a matter of pride this can get me in trouble. I should go through that without getting angry. I have done this before and I can do it again.

Finally, I hope it has become crystal clear the critical relationship between mindset and physical health – that mindset really defines and destines physical health status.

ABOUT THE AUTHOR

Amira Elshalaby, MSc. MA

Psychologist, nutritionist, psychotherapist, CBT therapist, psychotherapist counsellor, health and life coach, exercise nutrition coach (PN), personal trainer, personal stylist (basics), independent researcher, and professor via e-course creating and as a book author.

Academic journey

I obtained my first international diploma in Nutrition-Fitness at 18 years old and began my continuous academic international studies, as I have obtained more than 12 diplomas in Holistic Health/Medicine with grade A pass, Nutrition, Diet and Fitness, Human Health, Mental Health and in Psychology (clinical, abnormal, work organisation psychology, also in psychotherapy and counselling etc).

Finally, I obtained my MSc in Nutrition (public health, diet and weight loss etc.) and MA in Psychology (clinical, social psychology, health psychology etc.) in 2019 with a passing degree.

Along this long journey of academic studies and my own continuous self-research, I was always dedicating all my studies, knowledge, my vision, and understanding of health psychology science, other than my own vision of life, and personal experiences to help others try to be beneficial somehow to my surrounding society and people.

Since my real intention is to help people, that drives me to prioritise self-studying and researching more than making huge profits from being professional in one or certain profession(s). As I have found that working as a professor in a certain domain at whatever university would benefit limited people/students, the same as if I got a senior job in whatever significant company/organisation would hinder my main goal to make knowledge available to both the public and professionals and to reach and help the biggest number of people.

Also, it would disrupt my varied interests in learning languages such as French and Spanish, fashion jewellery styling, photography, interior design, etc. that I work on growing them as a great helper in my goal to help and impact wider people and to make their lives healthier, happier and thus of course wealthier.

So, I made my decision to write books right after obtaining my master's degrees, to share in transforming scientific info, valuable knowledge and represent my own understanding and vision of holistic health/medicine science to raise health awareness as an independent researcher and instructor via e-course creating, and writing books as I do now.

My motivation behind being willing to write books

I noticed that there is a common problem in the healthcare industry in this century is the tendency to gain huge profits in compensation for helping people and raising health awareness. Also, I found that many people including professionals lack the essential info that is needed to manage health status and thus life potential. This is due to either lack of awareness/info availability or lack of money to seek proper health care or training.

As a result, I intend to make my book(s) to combat such obstacles or boundaries since books or e-courses that are now available on the internet are so powerful and an easy, accessible method to provide and transfer valuable info related to health to people worldwide yearning to maintain their health,

This way, many people can be soldiered with info that assesses their problems, raises their health awareness so they can manage their health-life challenges, and make themselves more resilient and happier.

My mindset, my own life experience/knowledge and my positive mindset

My vision of life stems from my never-endless passion and energy to seek wisdom, gather valuable info and learn positive knowledge, and happy/healthy living methods in each and every way possible as this is my personality's core. Since I was a young child at 3-4 years old, I have had a philosopher's or analyst's way of thinking, therefore positive thinking/mindset is the basis of my life; it defines me and my life experience as I will now reveal.

My journey of accumulating knowledge and seeking wisdom was long and started at a very early age.

I have a unique experience in successfully and safely overcoming severe, tough and ambiguous problems that have detrimental health and life consequences in every moment of my life under ongoing very negative surroundings and circumstances with no professional help or even any kind of help or support. As such, the problems were not visible to anyone but me, its symptoms were not vibrant or detectable to either the public or professional which put me in a really miserable maze with no outlet or relief.

However, I was able to detect it even though I did not know its name or recognise scientifically its dimensions and definition. Although I was a little child, my vision and sense of rationality, science and health were never wrong. Then, as I reached 13 years old, its symptoms were quite vibrant only to me and really became a totally hidden paralysis to my body, mind, and soul.

I made myself my own researcher, psychologist, health professional and moreover an army leader, trying to find evidence that my detection and strategies were the right way to combat such disasters even though such damned problems were disabling me from doing any mental activities such as reading and learning. Of course, it was a lie and oppositely I followed my sense and thought that searching in ancient civilisation philosophy and health books, especially those that were available to me in my country (Egypt) at the time, for example, nutritional guides of the Ancient Egyptians (for the correlation between proper food intake and proper mental health) and Arab Muslim philosophers' books that summarise and analyse all the rationality and positive mindset sciences: philosophy, health science and psychology practices of their own and of the whole ancient world civilisations with personalised comments from the authors.

Thus, I succeeded in getting my evidence from my own miraculous research, then focused on the next step: how can I reach the current modern western scientific research that defines and treats such problems or even if there is any that discusses such problems to assure my conclusions or solutions?

While I was struggling to see the whole picture, I never stopped seeking, self-studying international courses via "distant mood" in varied arts of physical and mental health science as best as I could. Then, after many awful difficulties, I succeeded in discovering my awful problem's name and the best solution for it in the modern time we live in.

To recognise such a disaster's definition or name, I searched for it on the internet till I found research represented by a famous American psychologist (available to the public for a limited time). I considered his opinions, and treatment methods that luckily assured my vision, and then I committed to modern notices and strategies to enhance my health and recovery.

It was such a miraculous struggle to assess this disaster, as I did it by myself with no social or professional help just via my mind's vision, heart commitment, and self-research from ancient resources till I finally found modern evident research made for self-therapy as a published course on the internet. This took over 10 years, from when I was 12-23 years old.

In this way, I made a link between health psychology science in the past and the present (East-West civilisation) according to my own vision and my research that has never gone wrong since I was a little child. Of course, this journey was full of details, difficulties, and secrets that might need another book to explain.

However, I can summarise it in one way: I adhered faithfully and superstitiously to a positive mindset at all costs, even though it was impossible in such a problem that is characterised by making negative thinking patterns enter one's mind intrusively trying to dominate one's mind, heart, personality and thus life using one's power and beliefs. These drive them towards ongoing negativity and despair trying to make them ill in each moment and even more dangerously toward death (known as, social anxiety disorders).

Of course, such love, belief, and compliance to a positive mindset helped me conquer this incredibly awful and devastating problem safely saving my physical and mental health and more importantly to me, my identity, values, dignity, pride, peace, and happiness.

Thus, I realised from a very early age the power of the positive spirit and mind as the essence of health and life, which is the theme of this book *Mindset and Health*.

So, I hope that my book will be of great value to everyone who seeks better health and life.

Amira Elshalaby

ACKNOWLEDGEMENTS

The publishers and authors would like to thank Russell Spencer, Matt Vidler, Susan Woodard, Janelle Hope Leonard West, Lianne Bailey-Woodward, Laura Jayne Humphrey and Sakinah Richards for their work, without which this book would not have been possible.

ABOUT THE PUBLISHER

L.R. Price Publications is dedicated to publishing books by unknown authors. We use a mixture of both traditional and modern publishing options, to bring our authors' words to the wider world.
We print, publish, distribute and market books in a variety of formats including paper and hardback, electronic books, digital audiobooks and online.

If you are an author interested in getting your book published, or a book retailer interested in selling our books, please contact us.

www.lrpricepublications.com

L.R. Price Publications Ltd,
27 Old Gloucester Street,
London, WC1N 3AX.
020 3051 9572
publishing@lrprice.com

www.ingramcontent.com/pod-product-compliance
Lightning Source LLC
Chambersburg PA
CBHW060510280326
41933CB00014B/2914